Jesus slept. And so shoul
you to sleep – in a good
logical framework for res
eminently practical advi<

Josh Moody

Author of *Journey to Joy*, *No Other Gospel*, and *The God-Centered Life*
and Senior Pastor of College Church, Wheaton, Illinois

This is a dream book! It is a gentle, short read about something I love and would gladly spend ten hours a day doing if I could – sleeping. Read and discover how to honour God with your resting hours.

Krish Kandiah

Executive Director of Evangelical Alliance, Author of *Home for Good: making a difference for vulnerable children*
London

It's a delight to find this carefully biblical and engagingly personal treatment of a subject so vital to every human being. Adrian Reynolds has woven together Scripture's thematic threads on sleep in a way that both instructs and inspires thanksgiving to God for His providential ordering of our lives.

Kathleen B. Nielson

Director of Women's Initiatives, The Gospel Coalition,
Lookout Mountain, Georgia

Our attitudes to sleep are many and varied. Is it simply an inconvenience, stopping me getting more done in a busy life? Something we boast we can manage without? Or an idol to be worshipped? Something we pursue and cannot find and so worry about? And actually, is God even interested? The reality is our attitude to this significant part of our lives reveals something of our hearts and our attitude to our Creator. Written in a sensitive and conversational style, Adrian takes us through the biblical perspective on sleep. There's some great practical advice too. Read it! And thank God for the gift of sleep.

Anthony Adams
Church Planter and U.K. Director, Radstock Ministries, Derby

Some of us spend a third of our lives asleep; others wish we could. Adrian Reynolds writes to help us understand the principles of sleep and enjoy the practice. Beautifully written and biblically informed – this little volume makes… great bedtime reading.

Richard Underwood
Pastoral Director, The Fellowship of Independent Evangelical Churches, Market Harborough, England

As a husband, pastor and father of six young children I'm grateful to God for a good night's rest (when they come!). In this very readable book, Adrian Reynolds leads us through a study of what Scripture has to say about sleep so that we might embrace and enjoy this good gift that God has created for us, and in doing so have renewed hope in Him, as our heads hit the pillow. I'd encourage you to read it and be refreshed.

Nathan Smith
Lead Pastor
Grace Church, Bristol

With sleep problems being so common, it is refreshing to read a book that focuses on the spiritual and not just the medical side of this very important topic. Adrian walks us through what the Bible teaches about sleep and challenges us to apply these truths to our lives. A great little read which should make us turn to God and not just the pill box for a good night's sleep!

Matthew Sweeting
Locum Consultant Physician, Guy's and St. Thomas' NHS Foundation Trust. Part time church worker
Christ Church, Leyton

AND SO TO BED...

A biblical view of sleep

ADRIAN REYNOLDS

Adrian Reynolds is Director of Ministry of the Proclamation Trust and also serves as associate minister at East London Tabernacle Baptist Church.

Copyright © Adrian Reynolds 2014

paperback ISBN 978-1-78191-367-3
epub ISBN 978-1-78191-379-6
Mobi ISBN 978-1-78191-380-2

Published in 2014
by
Christian Focus Publications, Ltd.
Geanies House, Fearn, Ross-shire,
IV20 1TW, Scotland, United Kingdom.
www.christianfocus.com

Cover design by Daniel van Straaten

Printed by
Bell and Bain, Glasgow

CONTENTS

For Alice Deborah Clare

May your sleep be sweet
Proverbs 3:24

And so to bed
SAMUEL PEPYS, DIARIST
(Entry: 4 Jan. 1660)

START HERE

I have no Christian books on sleep.
I've plenty that *send me* to sleep, but that's not quite the same thing.

It's true. I've no Christian books on my shelf that give a biblical insight into this most important of subjects. Neither can I find any in my Christian bookstore, nor online. My *Dictionary of Pastoral Theology* (usually a great help) has no entry for sleep. It goes straight from 'slavery' to 'social contract'. Given the size of the problem and that sleep, as I hope to show you, is a spiritual issue, I found this all somewhat surprising.

As a pastor, I feel we're missing something. As a human being, I know we are.

There are plenty of us for whom 'good night' is something of a dream.

WHAT THIS BOOK IS

So, this little volume is my attempt to at least correct the imbalance in some measure. I want to tell you what the Bible has to say about sleep. Some of it may surprise you. Sleep is of greater spiritual importance than you may have imagined, both in terms of what it does for us now, but also in terms of what it teaches us about the future.

I'll start out by introducing sleep in general terms. Then I'll spend the bulk of the book trying to show you biblically my big idea:

> Sleep is part of our created humanity, a good gift from God to be treasured and enjoyed; an earthly picture of a spiritual reality.

Once I've done that, I'll spend just a little time explaining why it may be that some of us don't sleep all that well. What can we do – spiritually speaking – to help us sleep better?

There. That's it.

Now, at this point, you could just close the book. In one sense, I've nothing more to show you than this foundational description outlined above. But I hope you'll read on, because behind these simple twenty-four words are profound and encouraging truths.

My overall aim is to be both biblical and practical. Wonderfully, I don't believe these are, ultimately, different goals. God has made us in His image and we are whole people. We are not angels – spiritual beings without physical bodies. Nor are we simply collections of atoms and molecules. No, we have a soul, something which differentiates us from all of the rest of creation. As we shall see, though we share the need for sleep with much of the created world, there is more to it for us, for we are human beings made in the image of God.

WHAT THIS BOOK IS NOT

It's worth pointing out what this book is not, just so that you won't be disappointed. First, it's a book about sleep but it's not a book about dreams. The two are connected in some ways and the whole question of dreaming also represents an enormous biblical topic with significant theological implications. However, I don't want to cloud the important issue of sleep with too much talk of the more glamorous subject of dreams. So, if you're hoping for a book on the visions of the night, I'm sorry, you'll have to look elsewhere.

Second, it's a book about sleep but it's not a medical book. It is a book about the Bible's view of sleep and – to some extent – the Bible's remedy for sleeplessness. I will touch, very briefly, on medical and environmental issues to do with sleep, but this is not really a book about them. Please hear me carefully. There may well be health reasons why you struggle to sleep. There may also be environmental issues. I am neither a doctor nor a sleep counsellor, and all I can do is to point you in the right direction for help.

So, I'm not claiming that biblical answers are the only answers. But I do assert that we may often – perhaps too often – overlook what the Bible has to say about such an important subject.

SOME THANK-YOUS

It's right for an author to acknowledge the help he's received. So here goes. But, just to say, I won't be offended if you skip this bit and move swiftly on.

I've spent the last twenty-two years of my life sleeping with someone else in my bed. My beautiful wife, Celia, has not only been my life partner, but my sleep partner. It's helped. I want to thank God for her.

We have three daughters, but this particular issue of sleep has been one we've especially wrestled with as our eldest daughter has gone through various health issues. Her hard-won battles in every area of life have encouraged me to think about this subject biblically and this little volume is dedicated to her, with a father's love.

Some years ago now, I heard a sermon on sleep by C.J. Mahaney.[1] I confess that I now remember very little of it, but it started my thinking and research and so I gratefully acknowledge my debt.

Friends in ministry also serve (or have served) as family doctors and I'm especially grateful to Dr Rebecca Scott for helping me with chapter 5 and for reading through the final manuscript. I'm also grateful for colleagues (in particular Christopher Ash and Tim Ward) who have been unfailingly cheeky ('Can I write a book on coffee next?') but have sacrificially found time to read the book and helped me improve it, both biblically and pastorally. I am also indebted to John van Eyk, minister of the Tain/Fearn congregation of the Associated Presbyterian Church for his insightful help.

Finally, I am, of course, enormously thankful to, and dependent upon, the Living God – the One who never slumbers or sleeps.

He is the reason I can.

---

1. Available from www.sovereigngracestore.com by searching for 'sleep'.

1

NIGHT NIGHT!

Introducing sleep

Sleep. We all need it. We all do it.
We all – at some point – struggle with it.

Few people can disagree with these three statements. I'm perhaps one of the lucky ones. For much of my life I've been a good sleeper. I've never worked night shifts, and I've generally had regular patterns of waking and sleeping. However, despite this, there have been painful times when sleep has eluded me. And I know I'm not alone. Anecdotally, all my friends have – from time to time (and some more regularly than others) – struggled to get to sleep.

'The main facts in life are five,' said novelist E.M. Forster. 'Birth, food, sleep, love and death.'[1] Birth and death we can do little about. They have

---

1.   E.M. Forster, *Aspects of the Novel* (London, UK: Penguin, 2005).

their appointed times and occur only once for each member of humanity. Food and love are – to some extent – within our control. At least, we think they are. But what about sleep?

Instinctively, we know we need it (an instinct I hope to show is both medically and biblically appropriate). And we also know the frustration of missing out or, worse still, finding sleep impossible.

> A flock of sheep that leisurely pass by
> one after one; the sound of rain, and bees
> murmuring, the fall of rivers, winds and seas,
> Smooth fields, white sheets of water, and pure sky –
> I've thought of all by turns, and still I lie
> sleepless;
>> (William Wordsworth, *To sleep*, 1806)

We might, perhaps, have not expressed our difficulties in quite so poetic a manner as dear old Willie. Nevertheless, surveys repeatedly confirm what he rather romantically describes: we struggle with sleep.

IT'S A PROBLEM. REALLY.

In 2011, The Mental Health Foundation in the UK conducted one of the largest sleep surveys ever undertaken.[2] They asked people to assess their sleep on a score of 0–100 per cent, 100 per cent being a perfect night's sleep. The results were alarming.

The average sleep scores were 61 per cent for men and 57 per cent for women. This dropped below 50 per cent for those over 60. Of all those

---

2. For a full breakdown of the findings, see www.howdidyousleep.org.

surveyed, only 38 per cent were classified as 'good sleepers'. An extraordinary 36 per cent were classified as having possible chronic insomnia, a condition which involves serious sleep deprivation 'for a period of four weeks or more'.[3]

Interestingly, those who complained of a lack of sleep highlighted the effect this had on a variety of life issues, including:

- Difficulty maintaining healthy relationships.

- Low mood during the day.

- Difficulty staying awake during the day.

You will not be surprised at these findings. The difficulties will differ in their effect: a desk worker may not work particularly well following a sleepless night but he or she is unlikely to do anything more serious than fall asleep at the desk. A pilot, or bus driver, however…. You can see where this is going. Sleeplessness is more than an inconvenience. It is potentially deadly.

In the U.S.A., according to SleepCottage, 20 per cent of all motor vehicle accidents are caused by people falling asleep at the wheel. Doctors, they say, with less than six hours' sleep between procedures make *double* the rate of surgical errors.[4] Whether these data are accurate or not is hardly the point; we all *suspect* they might well be.

Why? Because most of us, I guess, have at some point experienced at least something of this

---

3. This is the definition used by a U.K. Private Health Provider, Bupa.

4. See www.sleepcottage.com.

sleeplessness and its effect. Everyone's been grumpy after a night of tossing and turning. Or worse.

It's easy, of course, to laugh off a lack of sleep. Perhaps that's our default position. Some people even wear it as a badge of honour. Bertrand Russell, the great British essayist, said, 'Men who sleep badly... are nearly always proud of the fact.'[5] Perhaps he is overstating his case. But we've all met people who like you to know how badly they've slept, as though it is some kind of macho qualification.

The truth is, we're often in awe of those who seem to need little sleep. The BBC reports that Napoleon, Florence Nightingale and Margaret Thatcher all got by on four hours' sleep a night.[6] (This is probably the only thing they had in common!). That makes complaining about a lack of sleep all seem a bit...well, weak and feeble. A recent article in *The Spectator* magazine highlighted this as a particular problem in modern America:

> Our war on sleep is hard to miss . TV interviewers ask today's hard-driving inventors how long they sleep...when the guest leaves, the interviewers bat the question around with each other, boasting about pulling 'all-nighters' in college or claiming 'I'm OK with five', revelling in a festival of one-downmanship. If the standard recommendation of eight hours a night gets mentioned, it is treated with genial contempt and the insistence that 'everybody's different'.[7]

5. Bertrand Russell, *The Conquest of Happiness* (London, UK: Routledge, 2006).

6. www.bbc.co.uk/science/humanbody/sleep.

7. Florence King, writing in *The Spectator* magazine p. 20 (London, UK: 25 January 2014).

Can that be right? In order to answer that question, we've got to delve a bit deeper and understand exactly what sleep is.

SLEEP LIKE A....SNAKE

On our last family holiday we visited the Cotswold Wildlife Park. I have to confess that the reptile house (which always promises much) was a trifle disappointing. Especially the snakes. The park owns an enormous reticulated python. And I mean *enormous*. Its thickness around was thicker than my youngest daughter's waist, which made me rather glad of the protective glass barrier.

But here's the thing about the python. It was quite dull to watch. Sure, its size impressed me. But it was coiled up in the corner, immovable. Researching for this book, I've now discovered why that is. The python sleeps for eighteen hours in every day. The chances of your visiting and seeing it move are pretty slim.

On the other hand, giraffes need only two hours' sleep in every day. And true to form, the giraffes were a much better spectator attraction. On your next zoological visit, I recommend you head there first.

Every living creature needs to sleep. There's great variation (as it happens, pythons and giraffes pretty much represent the two extremes). Some animals even take things further, of course. Hibernation is the name given to the reduced metabolic state that some creatures use to shut down over winter. It is extremely efficient at reducing the body's need for those things which generally keep them alive.

Those who crave sleep may be disappointed to hear it is not normal for humans to hibernate, although in 1900 the *British Medical Journal* reported the curious case of peasants in the Pskov region of Russia:

> At the first fall of snow the whole family gathers around the stove, lies down, ceases to wrestle with the problems of human existence, and quietly goes to sleep. Once a day everybody wakes up to eat a piece of hard bread. The members of the family take it in turn to watch and keep the fire alight. After six months of this reposeful existence the family wakes up, shakes itself and goes out to see if the grass is still growing and, by and by, sets to work at summer tasks.[8]

As *the New Statesman* wryly commented, 'the author has rather a sunny view of things... I can't believe the Russians leapt so cheerily to their feet.'[9] Such hibernation is not normal. But sleep is.

For humans, the amount of sleep also varies from person to person but the variations depend mainly on age. On average, newborn babies need about 16–18 hours' sleep. This decreases to 13–14 hours' sleep after about one year. (I can already hear some mums crying out, 'Why doesn't my Timmy sleep that much?', to which the answer is, he probably does if you stop to add it up. It often just doesn't *feel* like it.)

---

8. BMJ 2000;320:1245.2, cited in *The Times* newspaper p. 52 (London, U.K.: 10 December 2013).

9. Sophie Elmhirst writing in the *New Statesman* 27 February 2012, accessed online.

Children need less sleep – approximately 9–10 hours – and teenagers one hour less again (though you might think they would actually *like* much more if you've ever tried to get them out of bed in the morning). Most adults require 7–8 hours' sleep and older adults can get by on 6–7 hours, though this is supplemented (as you may know!) by naps during the day.

Let's make that real. If you are an average kind of adult and you go to bed at 11p.m. and it takes you half an hour to nod off, that means you should be waking at around 7.30 a.m. If your workday means you have to be up and about by 6.30 a.m., you should be heading to bed between 10 and 11p.m.

Put that way, many of our night-time sleep patterns might seem a little deficient. No wonder our sleep scores are so low.

Sleep metaphors have even entered our language. We talk of 'sleeping like a baby' although, as some wit has pointed out, anyone who uses that expression probably doesn't *have* a baby. Anyway, we might add, what does it mean to sleep like a baby? Do you wake up every two hours crying for food? Of course not: the phrase simply reflects the relatively long and uninterrupted sleep that most babies (over a few months old) need and enjoy.

What is it about sleep that is so important? Doesn't sleep just get in the way of a good time? Isn't sleep the thing we do when we've exhausted all other avenues for a top night out? Isn't Virginia Woolf, the famous author, correct when she says, 'Sleep is that deplorable curtailment of the joy of life'?[10]

---

10. Taken from Woolf's essay *Montaigne.*

OH RATS!

The answer, scientifically at least, is no. She's not right. Without sleep, there would be no joy of life, no good times and no cracking nights out. Scientists estimate that – were such an experiment possible – you would die of lack of sleep before you died of lack of food. We cannot function without proper sleep.

You can observe this by conducting sleep studies with rats. Such studies are less common now due to animal welfare objections. However, in the past, scientists have observed that sleep-deprived rats soon die. By placing rats on a small platform above water, the rat is deprived of sleep. It's still provided with food and water, it just can't snooze. Each time it nods off, the rat loses its balance and falls into the water, shocking it into wakefulness. Soon, the rat dies.

The results of this kind of research are largely discredited today because scientists cannot be sure whether it is the lack of sleep or the enormous stress that kills the rat first. Fair point. But the two are not unconnected, as anyone who has suffered lack of sleep knows – sleeplessness is stressful whether or not you are suspended above water.

Most scientists, however, would like to understand sleep better. It is relatively straightforward to observe, but more difficult to understand. It is still something of a medical mystery. One scientist has described the desire to understand why we sleep as 'the holy grail of sleep biology'.[11] As one of my

---

11. Steven Lockley & Russell Foster, *Sleep: a very short introduction* (Oxford, U.K.: OUP, 2012).

colleagues has dryly pointed out to me, given that they need so little sleep, it does make you wonder why giraffes are not ruling the universe.

To be a bit more technical (and more serious), there are approximately five measurable stages to sleep. (Scientists can measure these through observation and monitoring of brain activity.) Four of these are what clever types call non-REM sleep (where REM stands for rapid-eye-movement). One stage is REM sleep. In each night's sleep (assuming it's a good one), we go through four or five cycles of non-REM and REM sleep – back and forth, back and forth.

Non-REM sleep stages include drifting off to sleep (often accompanied by sudden body movement), slowing of breathing and heart rate, and moving into what we normally call deep sleep. These are all non-REM kinds of sleep. Then there is REM sleep, so called because it is distinguished by the movement of the eye (even when the eyes are closed). REM sleep is also part of the normal pattern of sleep and is when we often dream – or, at least, the stage from which we remember our dreams. It is not as deep a sleep as non-REM sleep. However, scientists believe it is this unique combination of different phases which makes sleep the restful thing it is.

If you've ever shared a bed with a spouse, or a bedroom with a friend or sibling, you may well recognise some of these stages. Ever felt that feeling of falling and being jerked awake or slept next to someone twitching? Sure, that's called hypnic jerk and is a regular feature of early non-REM sleep. It's not as odd as you thought.

All this is observable and describes the nature of sleep without really getting to the heart of what sleep is. For this, scientists rely on observing what happens to your body when you *don't* sleep. That's much easier than trying to work out what's going on inside you when you do.

Studies demonstrate that sleep-deprived adults suffer – according to University of Manchester neuroscientist Penelope Lewis – from hormonal imbalances, compromised immune functions and a drop in body temperature. That suggests, she says, that sleep plays a key role in body maintenance.[12]

But these effects are nothing compared to the psychological effects seen in sleep-deprived patients. Her list is frightening: 'moodiness, hallucinations, paranoia, poor memory, difficulty concentrating and impaired decision making'. We can all identify with something in this list. Pretty much everyone has experienced the day after a sleepless night before. And even if you don't remember being irritable, you can bet someone else does!

In the U.S., research published in 2011 showed that those who had less than six hours' sleep a night had a 50 per cent increase in risk of developing colorectal adenomas, precursors to cancer tumours.[13] In a study of 24,000 Japanese women reported in

---

12. Penelope Lewis, *The Secret World of Sleep* (New York, U.S.A.: Palgrave Macmillan, 2013).

13. Reported on www.sciencedaily.com based on a study reported in U.S. journal *Cancer* 11 Feb 2011 (online edition).

the *British Journal of Cancer*, those with fewer than six hours' sleep a night suffered a 40 per cent increase in incidence of breast cancer.[14]

The UK's Mental Health Foundation is clear. 'Sleep is as important to our bodies as eating, drinking and breathing, and is vital for maintaining good mental and physical health. Sleeping helps to repair and restore our brains and our bodies.'[15]

It works the other way too. For, strangely, a good night's sleep may also make us more creative. In their book *Sleep: a very short introduction*, two neuroscientists, Steven Lockley and Russell Foster, list a number of great breakthroughs or achievements that have come to people after a good long nap. Richard Wagner, they claim, used sleep both to inspire and to equip him for composition.

Which seems ironic really: those Wagner operas really do send me to sleep. Some of them last *days*!

In short, sleep is good.

Not surprisingly, a whole medical discipline has grown up around sleep, or, rather, the lack of it. Our local hospital is brand new. Built at a cost of several hundreds of millions of pounds, it has every facility you can imagine. I recently paid a visit to the neurological department there to accompany someone for a standard EEG test (an electroencephalogram, a test on brain activity). The floor of the hospital we visited also housed two sleep suites.

---

14. Reported on www.naturalnews.com based on a study reported in the *British Journal of Cancer* 23 Sept 2008 (online edition).

15. www.howdidyousleep.org.

These were not places for the staff to grab a quick afternoon nap (though I can't help wondering whether occasionally they may have been used that way), but, rather, therapy units to observe those with sleep problems and help patients overcome difficulties.

There is a whole range of sleep-related disorders, of varying degrees of seriousness, that have emerged over time: insomnia (inability to sleep); hypopnea (breathing difficulties during the night); sleep apnoea (obstruction of the airways during sleep); bruxism (teeth grinding); somnambulism (sleep-walking to you and me): all, and more, problems that the world recognises need to be fixed in some way.

Yes, in short, sleep is good and the whole world knows it.

That's the science, or at least the level of science that someone like me can understand. But what about the Bible? Is sleep a good thing in the Bible too? If sleep is such a hot topic, we would expect the Bible to say something about it, wouldn't we?

And it does. That's where we turn to next.

2

GOOD NIGHT!

Sleep is part of our created humanity

Jesus slept.

That unremarkable statement is more significant than we imagine. Both Matthew and Mark record the story of Jesus calming the storm. A key component of this brief but gripping story is that Jesus was asleep.

> Then he got into the boat and his disciples followed him. Suddenly a furious storm came up on the lake, so that the waves swept over the boat. But Jesus was sleeping. The disciples went and woke him, saying, 'Lord, save us! We're going to drown!' He replied, 'You of little faith, why are you so afraid?' Then he got up and rebuked the winds and the waves, and it was completely calm. The men were amazed and asked, 'What kind of

man is this? Even the winds and the waves obey
him!' (Matt. 8:23-27)

This must be one of the most well-known New
Testament stories. It's taught in Sunday schools and
on evangelistic Bible courses. It reveals, of course,
something of the identity of Christ Jesus. He is the
man whom even the winds and waves obey.

But do you notice what detail is integral to the
story? Whilst the waves broke over the boat and
the wind whipped the rigging into a frenzy, the
Son of God was soundly asleep. This is more, of
course, than a comment on Jesus' sea legs. The
disciples were serious mariners too and they were
certainly not asleep. Rather, it is about faith that
assures of safety. Jesus had this faith in His Father's
providential care. The disciples did not.

That tells us two things about sleep. First – and
this is the one we will concentrate on in this chapter
– sleep is part of our created humanity. Second –
and this is for the next chapter – the willingness to
lie down and sleep is itself an expression of trust
and faith in a sovereign God.

But first things first. Jesus slept.

Jesus is the perfect man. 'In him,' says the
Apostle John, 'is no sin' (1 John 3:5) a fact also
repeated by the Apostle Paul (2 Cor. 5:21) and
the Apostle Peter (1 Pet. 2:22). There is no doubt
that the sinlessness of Christ Jesus is a key part of
the Apostles' teaching. But we can say more than
this. Jesus' perfection was not just because He was
God Himself, but because He was the perfect man,
fulfilling (for example) the psalmist's vision of

humanity found in Psalm 8. 'He had to be made like them, fully human in every way, in order that he might become a merciful and faithful high priest in service to God, and that he might make atonement for the sins of the people' (Heb. 2:17, commenting on Ps. 8).

When we look at Jesus, therefore, we see the perfect man. That is brilliant news for us, for it is only as the perfect man that Jesus can be the perfect Saviour. We ought to rejoice in His humanity more! Evangelicals are sometimes a bit woolly on this. We know Jesus is fully God and we rejoice in this. However, keen as we are to get past the 'He was just a good man/teacher' objection to Christianity, we sometimes neglect to rejoice in His humanity.

So, little details, like the one in our passage in Matthew, pass us by. Jesus slept.

Here is the perfect man, tired and needing rest. Nor can we say this is just a detail to make the story more significant. No; elsewhere, we read of Jesus getting tired. This is the reason for His rest at the well where he meets the Samaritan woman: 'Jacob's well was there and Jesus, tired as he was from the journey, sat down by the well' (John 4:6).

It's normal to be tired. And it's normal to need sleep.

Sure, there are occasional times when it is also right to stay awake. Jesus got up early to pray (Mark 1:35) and stayed awake in the Garden of Gethsemane whilst His disciples succumbed to their drowsiness (Mark 14:37). But these occurrences shouldn't detract from the normal pattern.

Sleep, on this basis, is not something to be denied or decried. We shouldn't listen to those who mock sleep, nor give any weight to those who see lack of sleep as a badge of honour. 'I stayed up all night working,' my university friends used to boast to me. There's nothing big and clever in that. I must confess, in my previous working life, to once staying up all night (photocopying, if you must know). But it was pointless. I couldn't do any work the next day and we lost the legal case for which we had been preparing anyway.

No, sleep is a normal part of our created humanity. Everyone gets tired, as the Scriptures acknowledge. 'Even youths grow tired and weary, and young men stumble and fall' (Isa. 40.30).

Remarkably, in Jesus, we see not only a pattern of sleep, but a concern that others should enjoy the same kind of rest. There's a wonderfully moving statement at the beginning of the story of the feeding of the five thousand which reveals Jesus as the compassionate leader. 'Because so many people were coming and going that they did not even have a chance to eat, he said to them, "Come with me by yourselves to a quiet place and get some rest."'(Mark 6:31). And so they did.

SLEEPING OUTSIDE?

Was there sleep in the Garden of Eden, then, right at the beginning of history? Did sleep exist before sin did?

Sleep is certainly mentioned in Genesis 1–2. But it is not so much a rest from work or a daily nap as a divinely imposed surgical anaesthesia where God puts Adam into a deep sleep so woman can be made from him (Gen. 2:21). 'So the LORD God caused the man to fall into a deep sleep.'

Perhaps, in the light of our thinking about Jesus, we could say that there *was* sleep in the garden. Jesus is the perfect man even though He lived in a broken world. In one sense, He felt the effects of the sin around him – He saw illness and felt the pain of the death of a friend, for example. His own death on our behalf arose as a result of the sinfulness and evil in the world, both as a remedy for it (He died *for* us), but also caused by it (He was put to death by sinful men).

But there is nothing to suggest in the Scriptures that this sinfulness affected His person. It could not. He was and is sinless. The first Adam shared, initially, this characteristic. He would have needed sleep too. As would Eve.

Some people would like to argue that sleep is just another aspect of Jesus, the eternal Son of God, becoming flesh and being 'numbered with the transgressors' (Isa. 53:12). We can't be certain, they would say, but it is possible that sleep is a consequence of the brokenness of the world in which we live. Given the overwhelmingly positive way sleep is described in the Scriptures, I think this is unlikely.

Either way, we still see a need to sleep in Jesus. We see Him enjoying the good gift that sleep is.

All this brings us to an interesting, though, it must be admitted, less than essential thing to say about sleep in the Scriptures. The Old Testament, in particular, has many words for sleep. Our translations tend to soften the vocabulary, which is richer than you may think. There is a word for a lighter sleep and there is a word for a deeper sleep. There is even (and we shall think about this later in the book) a word which means 'to be shut up'. That's the equivalent of us saying 'go out like a light' – meaning to drop into a very deep sleep.

There's a word for lying down, which is often translated sleep (though not always – perhaps most famously in Psalm 23:2: 'He makes me lie down in green pastures.'). The Bible recognises, in other words, the variety of sleep that scientists now understand. Bible writers knew from experience that sleep is sometimes deep, sometimes not.

HEAVENLY SLEEP

What about the future? If there is sleep in the Garden, will there be sleep in the new creation? The Bible is silent on this – like much of the detail of the New Jerusalem to come. There's part of me that hopes so. I *do* like sleep, and I would rather like to think that sleep will be in the new creation, *only even better*.

But though our humanity continues on into the new creation, it does change. Jesus retains His humanity but now sits at the right hand of the Father, 'sustaining all things by his powerful word' (Heb. 1:3). There doesn't seem to be much room there for sleep! His sustaining rule is uninterrupted on into eternity. Jesus needed sleep in His earthly humanity, a need we now share. If, in His perfect glorified humanity, He does not need sleep, it seems reasonable to assume that we too will not need to go to bed every night.

And to those who want to say that sleep is a part of our created humanity and therefore *must* continue into the new creation, we need to say that the Scriptures teach that some things *will* change. The new creation is not simply a return to Eden. At its most fundamental, there Adam and Eve were *able* to sin. In the new creation, we can categorically say, there will be no more sin.

Paul knows this step change will take place and explains it to his Corinthians friends.

> If there is a natural body, there is also a spiritual body....The spiritual did not come first, but the natural, and after that the spiritual. The first man was of the dust of the earth, the second man is of heaven. As was the earthly man, so are those who are of the earth; and as is the heavenly man, so also are those who are of heaven. And just as we have borne the image of the earthly man, so shall we bear the image of the heavenly man. (1 Cor. 15:44-49)

Paul is clear in this chapter of 1 Corinthians that the resurrection body is not natural, it is spiritual. He does not mean that it is all floaty and ghost-like. No, the resurrection body is still physical, just as that of Jesus was. Jesus' resurrection body could be touched by His followers. He ate a meal with them by the side of the lake. And yet there was a fundamental change between His pre-resurrection body and His post-resurrection one. That is what Paul is explaining here.

There is a change from natural to spiritual. The spiritual body is not bound by the earthly limitations placed upon it. Jesus could pass through a locked door! It seems to me, therefore, that this means sleep may be something we do not need in the new creation. Heaven is not one long lie-in!

Better enjoy sleep now then.

Which brings us neatly to the next chapter.

3

SLEEP TIGHT!

Sleep is a good gift to be treasured and enjoyed

Nobody likes to be woken in the middle of a good sleep. The comedian Steve Martin says that the best way to get sincere advice and an accurate time check is to ring any number at random in the middle of the night.[1] (Think about it... 'Do you realise what time it is....?') That's because, without really needing to be told (and as we've already seen), we know that sleep is good; it does us good. We don't appreciate it being disturbed.

Everybody has had that feeling when they wake up after a good night's sleep and feel refreshed and ready. And I hope you've had it pretty recently!

Remember, we've been building up a biblical picture of sleep. This is where we will ultimately end up:

---

1. Recorded in David Young, *Great Funny Quotes* (Round Rock, Texas, U.S.A.: Wind Runner Press, 2011).

Sleep is part of our created humanity, a good gift from God to be treasured and enjoyed; an earthly picture of a spiritual reality.

True, we've not, as yet, got very far into our definition. However, what we've looked at so far is important foundational stuff. Now, things start to get interesting. It shouldn't surprise us that if sleep is part of our created humanity, it's actually *a good thing*. Our heavenly Father is the giver of every good and perfect gift (James 1:17), and that must include sleep, mustn't it?

Well, if so, we would expect it to be explicit in the Bible. And guess what? It is. Listen to the words of King Solomon:

Unless the LORD builds the house, the builders labour in vain.

Unless the LORD watches over the city, the guards stand watch in vain.

In vain you rise early and stay up late, toiling for food to eat –

For he grants sleep to those he loves.

(Ps. 127:1-2)

Now, before we get into what this psalm teaches us about sleep, we've got to clear up one thing. Your Bible footnote may hint that there is more than one way to read this psalm. It may suggest that an alternative ending goes something like 'For while they sleep he provides food.'

What did King Solomon really mean when he wrote this psalm? In technical terms, it all turns on the translation of a particularly tricky word. However, for our purposes, it is enough to see that Solomon is looking to paint a contrast between the man or woman who trusts in their own work and abilities and the one who trusts in God. In this context, sleep (as most Bible versions recognise) is an appropriate translation: the ultimate picture of trusting God is being able to get your head down at night.

On this basis, we can see that sleep is a gift from God.

FANCY A LIE-DOWN?

David confirms this in his well-known shepherding psalm:

> The LORD is my shepherd, I lack nothing.
>
> He makes me lie down in green pastures,
>
> he leads me beside quiet waters. (Ps. 23:1-2)

In this context, 'lie down' can only mean sleep. According to *sheep101.info* (the web's 'beginner's guide to sheep'!), sheep only lie down to sleep or rest. Everything else (including giving birth) is done from a standing position. It's clear, therefore, what David means. The LORD, his shepherd, is the one who gives him rest and sleep. It's a gift.

This truth is backed up by the fact that Asaph tells the negative side of the story. In Psalm 77 (a song we shall return to later), Asaph cannot sleep. We're going to discover why this is in the chapter after next (clue: there's an issue to be resolved). But for the moment, we need to see that his *lack of sleep* is also something God ordains.

> I remembered you, God, and I groaned;
> I meditated and my spirit grew faint.
> *You* kept my eyes from closing;
> I was too troubled to speak. (Ps. 77:3-4)

If it is God who prevents us from sleeping (for a particular purpose), it follows that it is also He who gives sleep in the first place.

Of course, some would want to say that sleep comes to us for all kinds of physical reasons: we are tired; we have worked hard; it's late, and so on. All true. But the physical realities need not hide the spiritual truth: sleep is a gift.

We know, for example, the scientific reasons that a plant grows. We know how it gets from the field to the table (or, at least, we have a pretty good idea). But no Christian denies that the food on our tables is a good gift from our heavenly Father. And so it is with sleep.

But we can say more.

Sleep is not just a gift. It is a *good* gift.

Sleep is not always mentioned positively in the Bible (and we shall see a few instances where that is the case later). But, in the right context, the Bible is overwhelmingly positive about sleep. The Creator's word – if you like – backs up what the scientists have discovered later. Sleep is a good thing.

SWEET AND PLEASANT
One of my favourite proverbs comes near the beginning of that remarkable book:

My son, do not let wisdom and understanding out of your sight,

preserve sound judgment and discretion;....

When you lie down, you will not be afraid;

when you lie down, your sleep will be sweet. (Prov. 3:21, 24)

The one who fears God and keeps His commands is the one, in New Testament terms, who follows, loves and serves Christ Jesus, the Wisdom of God. And if we live without letting go of the sight of Jesus, here is a remarkable statement: we will not be afraid when we sleep; indeed our sleep will be sweet.

We'll come back to the first of those points shortly. For now, I want you to see the wonderful way that sleep is described in the proverb. It is something that is sweet. Sweet means good. Sweet means nice. Sweet means wonderful. Sweet means great to taste. And more.

We often say to our young children, 'Sweet dreams', meaning "I hope you don't have any nightmares." We want them (and ourselves!) to sleep soundly through the night. In fact, if we had been a bit more savvy, we ought to say, 'Sweet *sleep*', for that is then using a Bible word to describe a Bible gift.

The prophet Jeremiah is troubled with many hard things that he must say to the people of Israel. They're not particularly good listeners, as you will know if you've read his prophecies. However, there's one wonderful moment when he dreams of a restored Israel: farms producing food; women giving birth; towns flourishing, and so on. Then Jeremiah awakes. This is what he records:

> At this I awoke and looked around. My sleep had been pleasant to me. (Jer. 31:26)

Do you notice what he said? Not 'my *dreams* had been pleasant' but 'my *sleep* had been pleasant.' His sweet dreams had made his sleep sweet.

Sleep is a good gift.

REMEMBER TO SAY THANK YOU

Which ought to make us pause and ask some searching questions. Is this a gift you ever pray for? Or thank God for?

The former is perhaps more natural than the latter. That is because we are better – in general – at asking for things than thanking God for them. But here's a challenge: when was sleep last a topic for praise? Perhaps if you've struggled to sleep that may focus the mind, but how many mornings do you wake up after a good night, stretch and cry out, 'Thank you, Lord, for the good gift of sleep'?

My wife and I pray together every night before we turn out the light. We thank God for the day, pray for tomorrow and for our children and then work our way systematically through the church prayer diary. Usually, I remember to pray for a good night's sleep. I'm more likely to do that if we've had trouble sleeping.

But I cannot remember, to my shame, ever waking in the morning and saying 'thank you'. My point is simple: if we really reckoned on sleep being a good gift from God, we would certainly be more thankful for it.

Any good gift should be treasured. But every good gift should also be enjoyed. In the sometimes perplexing book of Ecclesiastes, Solomon (yes, him again) teaches his people to make the most of what God gives. This world, he shows, is sometimes hard to fathom. Things don't always make sense. Sometimes they seem a little topsy-turvy. What is the best way to live in this kind of world? Number one: 'fear God and keep his commandments' (Eccles. 12:13). Or, to put it in New Testament language, walk closely with Jesus: trust *then* obey, we might say.

And number two? 'I commend the enjoyment of life' (Eccles. 8:15). Take the good things God has given and, in their proper context, enjoy them. That includes sleep. Here's the good news about sleep. It is not just a good gift for which we must thank God but one we ought to enjoy.

Rather than being embarrassed about a good night's sleep, we ought to rejoice in it. I mentioned to someone that I was writing a book about sleep. They were somewhat bemused. 'Why not write a book about going to the lavatory?' was the cheeky reply. The answer is because sleep is more than body functionality; it is a good gift to be *actively* treasured. It is a sweet, pleasant, good gift from our Father.

WHO'S AFRAID OF THE BIG BAD WOLF?
However, those words of Solomon hint at something even more profound about sleep. It is not just

39

a good gift to be treasured and enjoyed. I hope you agree with me on that. It is also a mark of something else. It is a sign of trust.

Did you notice how Solomon passed on his wisdom?

> My son, do not let wisdom and understanding out of your sight,
>
> preserve sound judgment and discretion;....
>
> When you lie down, you will not be afraid;
>
> when you lie down, your sleep will be sweet. (Prov. 3:21, 24)

How is it that Solomon can encourage us to lie down and not be afraid?

Monday night in our house is the night Dad is responsible for putting our youngest daughter to bed. We read, chat, pray and then (eventually) it's time for goodnight. In our house, this is a complex ritual which means that certain lights have to be turned on, others extinguished and doors left open a precise amount. It may be my lack of practice which means I often seem to get it wrong!

What's that routine all about? Ultimately, it is about making sure things are just right for my little daughter so she can sleep soundly. She wants to be safe, and there are certain routines and settings which give her that sense of security. Even into adulthood, many of us carry on the same kind of routines. I double-lock the door and set the alarm before going to bed every night.

Humanly speaking, if we are to sleep soundly, we have to trust certain things. I have to trust that the house is weatherproof and burglar-resistant. I trust the roof will not leak and the front door will stay shut. More immediately, I trust that the bed will hold me up through the night and the ceiling joists will hold so I don't wake in the morning to find myself in the living room, one floor down in our Victorian town house.

All of this we take for granted, but we must all acknowledge it's true.

The same is also true spiritually. We perhaps don't feel this as keenly as the Bible writers did They often slept outside and many of the psalmists, for example, faced dangers we can only imagine: wild animals, enemies and traitors.

In this context, sleep is always a mark of trust that we will be all right. In wartime, a guard is posted and soldiers take turns at keeping watch precisely because they cannot guarantee this kind of safety.

It's significant, therefore, that this is the way Bible writers speak about sleep. We've already seen what Solomon said. He may well have learnt the lesson from his dad, David. Read through these two examples:

> I lie down and sleep;
> I wake again, because the LORD sustains me.
> I will not fear though tens of thousands
> assail me on every side. (Ps. 3:5-6)

David wrote this whilst fleeing from his son Absalom, who was out to get him. Or what about this:

> In peace I will lie down and sleep,
>
> for you alone, LORD
>
> make me dwell in safety. (Ps. 4:8)

In both instances, David can sleep because he trusts in God's providential care. He is able – even though in battle situations – to sleep soundly because he knows God is with him, more than this, 'sustaining' him.

We could perhaps express it like this: the willingness to lie down and sleep is itself an expression of trust in the sovereign hand of God. Nothing is going to happen to me that He does not determine. Nothing bad is going to happen that He does not allow. Every breath I take is down to Him, waking or sleeping.

This peace about *going* to sleep expresses a trust and confidence that God is in control and watching over us. As the translation of the Old Irish hymn says:

> Lord, be my vision, supreme in my heart,
>
> bid every rival give way and depart:
>
> you my best thought in the day or the night,
>
> waking or sleeping, your presence my light.[2]

This brings us back full circle to the disciples panicking in the boat whilst Jesus slept – the story with which we

---

2.   Translated from the Poem Book of the Gael by Mary E. Byrne, selected and edited by Eleanor Hull (1860-1935). This version is from the *Praise!* hymnbook, number 732 (Darlington, U.K.: Praise Trust, 2000).

opened the last chapter. You can now see something of its significance. Jesus, the perfect man, can sleep because of His confidence in His heavenly Father. He knew He would not drown. This was not His time.

The disciples did not understand this. And so Jesus' rebuke is just the right one: 'You of little faith, why are you so afraid?' (Matt. 8:26).

INTRODUCING THE ONE WHO DOES NOT SLEEP
Ultimately, this truth is expressed in one of the most moving Scriptural passages that talks about sleep. In fact, to be more precise, it speaks of *not sleeping*. I am talking about Psalm 121:

> [1]I lift up my eyes to the mountains –
> where does my help come from?
> [2]My help comes from the Lord,
> the Maker of heaven and earth.
> [3]He will not let your foot slip –
> He who watches over you will not slumber;
> [4]indeed, he who watches over Israel
> will neither slumber nor sleep.
> [5]The Lord watches over you –
> The Lord is your shade at your right hand;
> [6]the sun will not harm you by day,
> nor the moon by night.
> [7]The Lord will keep you from all harm –
> he will watch over your life;
> [8]The Lord will watch over your coming and going
> both now and for evermore.

These are beautiful words, aren't they? This psalm is a song of ascents: that means that it was a song sung by the people of God as they went up to Jerusalem to celebrate one of the main Jewish festivals. In other words, these were well-known lines.

They express perfectly what we've already seen: that we can sleep because of God's sovereign care. The LORD God is the One who watches over us; He is our shade. Perhaps, though, the most important thought this adds to what we've already seen is this: we can sleep because God does not.

The language is wonderfully poetic. 'He who watches over Israel will neither slumber nor sleep.' Here are two of our sleeping words from Hebrew. The word translated 'slumber' is a word we might translate 'nod off'. It means drowsiness. God will not fall asleep at the wheel, so to speak. My father-in-law often tells me he's 'just closing his eyes'. That means he's taking his afternoon power nap.

Not God. He needs no afternoon nap.

It may also help you to know that the word translated 'sleep' in verse 4 is the more common Hebrew word meaning a proper sleep! I rather like the way Eugene Peterson renders it in his popular paraphrase: 'Not on your life! Israel's Guardian will never doze or sleep.'[3]

Here is the beautiful, wonderful, amazing, breath-taking paradox of sleep. We can sleep because He does not! It is precisely God's *sleeplessness* (or more

---

3. *The Message* translation.

exactly, His lack of need for sleep) that means our sleep can be safe, sound and tranquil.

God's sleepless character is the very reason that the good gift of sleep He gives to His children can be both treasured and enjoyed.

RIGHT PLACE, WRONG TIME

I hinted earlier that not everything the Bible says about sleep is positive. To be fair to the Bible's sweep, we have to pick out three particular exceptions.

First, we have to say that sleep, like all of God's good gifts, can easily become an idol. It is quite possible to love and desire sleep so much that the gift, rather than the Giver, becomes our focus. We should not be surprised at this danger.

Money, sex, security, family – all of these can easily become the things we desire above Christ; we can easily worship them. This is not just a general point: it is explicit in the Scriptures: 'do not *love* sleep or you will grow poor; stay awake and you will have food to spare' (Prov. 20:13). Now, it is important to understand the proverb in its context. It is warning against laziness. In a hand-to-mouth agricultural economy, if you don't work, you won't eat.

The proverb writer expresses this very memorably. 'Do not love sleep.' In other words, don't spend all day in bed – get up and do some work! Sleep here is an idol because it supplants the command to work. Nevertheless, the principle stands, even outside of the immediate context. Sleep can easily become an idol.

Which brings me to the next exception. Again, like all of God's gifts, it is the context which makes it good. We can see that most clearly in the gift of sexual intimacy. In its right context, it is a good and wonderful gift. In the wrong context, it is not a gift, but a sin. Most Christians are clear on this.

It is no different to sleep. There is a time to be awake. And sleeping at the waking time is just wrong. Although we do have the example of Eutychus falling asleep in a long sermon (Acts 20:7-12), I would suggest (as would most preachers) that falling asleep during sermons is not a good gift to be enjoyed and treasured. Try that line of argument with the pastor next time it happens!

Jesus makes this clear with His disciples who nodded off at the key moment in Gethsemane, the very time when He needed them most: 'Then he returned to his disciples and found them sleeping. "Couldn't you men keep watch with me for one hour?" he asked Peter' (Matt. 26:40). There was a time for them to be awake and this was it!

Then, finally, we need to be cautious lest we should ever think that the ability to sleep means everything is all right with us and our walk with Christ. There is the sleep of the righteous, as the saying goes, but it is also possible to sleep the sleep of the unrighteous.

To put it bluntly, the wicked sleep soundly too. It's possible to be living a life of rebellion against God and His purposes and still get a good night's kip. The best Bible example of this is Jonah. You probably know the story. God calls Jonah to go to Nineveh. But Jonah chooses instead to run off on a ship bound for Tarshish (pretty much in the opposite direction). The Lord sends a great storm.

But Jonah? He 'had gone below deck, where he lay down and fell into a deep sleep' (Jonah 1:5), an attitude which amazed the ship's captain. In this case, sleep was not a good gift to be treasured and enjoyed, but the mark of someone whose conscience was 'seared as with a hot iron' (1 Tim. 4:2).

These three exceptions are good to bear in mind. But none changes the general principle and truth: sleep is a good gift from our heavenly Father, a gift to be treasured and enjoyed. We can sleep because He doesn't.

No guarantees. Not yet, anyway.

Now, as this chapter draws to a close, we do have to be careful. The two psalms we quoted (Ps. 3 and Ps. 4) are Old Testament psalms rooted in the promises made in the Old Covenant to the Lord's anointed king, David. These Old Testament promises seem to be fixed on the here and now, but in fact are always pointing to a greater and deeper truth. To fully understand what God is promising we have to look beyond the immediate and see how promises made to the anointed kings are now fulfilled in Christ.

For example, the psalms express a confidence in God's protection. David could not have thought that he would always be free from his enemies. His experience taught him that was not so. Yet he was able to express a confidence in this life because he knew that – ultimately – the promise would always be proved to be true.

We see the same paradox in the words of Jesus. Some of His followers will be despised, even by

their families. Some will even be put to death
(Luke 21:16). They will be hated. And yet, Jesus
says, 'not a hair of your head will perish.' How so?

The answer is that because, even though we
cannot guarantee we will wake from our sleep safe
and sound every morning, we do have the certainty
of a greater promise. And that's what the next
chapter is about.

4

SEE YOU IN THE MORNING!

Sleep is an earthly picture of a spiritual reality

I live very near a cemetery. It might not sound very glamorous, but at least it means the neighbours are reasonably quiet. It is one of London's so-called super-cemeteries opened in the 1840s to deal with overcrowding in existing burial grounds. Most of the estimated 350,000 graves are unmarked, but one corner is given over to the graves of 'Dissenters' (non-Anglican Protestants). Reading some of the small, unassuming gravestones can be very moving. Victorian graves are like that; there are lots of graves of infants, small children and those who died young. Many of these Dissenters' tombstones are marked with three simple words: *asleep in Jesus*.

This is not Victorian political correctness. It's well known that modern Western societies have developed many alternative ways to describe death – some more coarse than others. We simply don't like to talk about death. And some might think that 'sleeping' is just another such euphemism.

But no. This is not that. These brothers and sisters were not afraid of death. They understood it. Those who died are asleep in Jesus.

DEAD OR ALIVE, PART ONE

That's not a new idea. It's a Bible one. Both Old and New Testaments use this as a way of describing death. It's less common in the Old Testament, but it's still there. As we've already seen, there are a number of different Hebrew words for death. One of them means, somewhat descriptively, to be stunned or closed; we might say 'go out like a light'. Our modern Bibles sometimes translate this word 'sleep' (Jonah 1:6, for example) and sometimes use it to describe death. 'The valiant lie plundered, they sleep their last sleep' (Ps. 76:5). I don't think there's any doubt what the psalmist Asaph means.

More clearly, in the New Testament, there is an obvious link between the language of sleep and the language of death. This is seen in the words of Jesus as He raises from the dead the daughter of Jairus.

'Stop wailing,' Jesus said. 'She is not dead but asleep.' They laughed at him, knowing that she was dead. But he took her by the hand and said, 'My child, get up!' Her spirit returned, and at once she stood up. (Luke 8:52-55)

We, the readers, are clear. We know she is dead. But notice how Jesus performs His reviving miracle using the language of sleep.

DEAD OR ALIVE, PART TWO

The very same thing happens in John 11. The story of Lazarus, the friend of Jesus, is familiar enough. It contains some very well-known moments and phrases, most notably, the wonderful words of the Saviour reassuring Martha that, 'I am the resurrection and the life. The one who believes in me will live, even though they die; and whoever lives by believing in me will never die' (John 11:25-26).

But rewind just a few moments and we get a startling insight as Jesus teaches His disciples.

> He went on to tell them, 'Our friend Lazarus has fallen asleep; but I am going there to wake him up.' His disciples replied, 'Lord, if he sleeps, he will get better.' Jesus had been speaking of his death, but his disciples thought he meant natural sleep. (John 11:11-13)

Just to clarify, Jesus then immediately makes it all more straightforward:

> So then he told them plainly, 'Lazarus is dead.' (v. 14)

Jesus seems to equate death with sleep because it implies that there is something more to come. The disciples do, at least, understand this about *sleep*. 'Lord, if he sleeps, he will get better.' But they seem not to understand this about *death*, something that

Martha *does* get: 'I know that he will rise again in the resurrection at the last day' (John 11:24).

DEAD OR ALIVE, PART THREE

Paul takes up this ambiguity and uses even more clearly the language of sleep to describe death.

> According to the Lord's word, we tell you that we who are still alive, who are left until the coming of the Lord, will certainly not precede those who have fallen asleep. (1 Thess. 4:15)

And lest there be any uncertainty about what Paul means here, he continues,

> For the Lord himself will come down from heaven, with a loud command, with the voice of the archangel and with the trumpet call of God, and *the dead in Christ* will rise first.

Why this confusion of language? Was the Apostle embarrassed about death and the language used to describe it, much like we might say someone has 'passed' or 'been lost'? Hardly. Elsewhere, he is pretty direct about death and its effects.

No. Rather, Paul knows that the language of sleep is eminently suitable to describe death. He is following the example of Jesus in describing death in this way.

Why is this the right language to use? Quite simply, it is because death is not the end.

The raising to life of Lazarus prefigured the resurrection of the Son of God. Death could not hold Him and, just as He had promised, He was raised to life on the third day. This wonderful and central truth, says the Apostle Paul, leads the way for what theologians sometimes call 'general resurrection' (meaning that it will happen more *generally*, i.e. to everyone). 'But Christ has indeed been raised from the dead, the first-fruits of those who have fallen asleep' (1 Cor. 15:20).

Because Christ was raised, so people will be raised too. The firstfruits are (as the name suggests) the first part of the harvest. They are important because they show you what kind of harvest you're going to get. If the first grapes are good, then the rest of the bunch will also be great. It's a moving description of Jesus' resurrection – pointing us towards what is in store for every believer.

Some like to think that death is the end, but as Christians we believe that death is simply a staging post on the way. To be joined to Christ means being made like Him in His death so that, to paraphrase Paul, we might be made like Him in His resurrection body. As the old French hymn puts it:

> It is not death to die,
> to leave this weary road,
> and midst the brotherhood on high
> to be at home with God.
>
> It is not death to close
> the eye long dimmed by tears,
> and wake, in glorious repose,
> to spend eternal years.[1]

---

1. This is an old nineteenth century French hymn by H. A. César Malan and translated by American Dutch Huguenot George W. Bethune. The full words are available at www.nethymnal.org/htm/i/i/n/iindeath.htm. A good modern version is available from Sovereign Grace Music.

Seen this way, sleep is a perfect analogy for death. Standing on the earthly side of eternity, death can seem very final. And, for sure, that is how it should be. Death breaks our link with this world. Our lifeless bodies are laid in the ground or cremated. Wills are proved. Assets distributed. For those left behind there is, certainly, a finality about death.

But as Christians we understand that this finality is only linked to this present world. Jesus' resurrection proves that the dead in Christ will also rise.

When we go to sleep, we fully intend to wake in the morning. We fully expect to nod off and then wake with the dawn. It's why we set alarm clocks, plan diaries, make appointments, and so on. No one goes to sleep thinking 'this will probably be it.' No, we expect that sleeping will be followed by waking, as sure as day follows night.

This is not true for everyone, of course. Sometimes death *does* take us in our sleep. Indeed, this is precisely the kind of death that some people hope will be their end. The idea of drawn-out illness and suffering is frightening. I've conducted funerals where the person being buried has died peacefully in their sleep. It's astounding how many relatives say something like 'That's the way I want to go too.'

The reality is that the 'way we go' is in the hands of our Sovereign God. For some, it may be a peaceful slipping away. For others, it may be a road marked with suffering. But, in both cases, sleep is the appropriate description of death.

EVERYONE WAKES UP

This is true, in fact, for both believers and unbelievers. The general resurrection applies to all: those who have died in Christ and those who have died rejecting Him. 'For we must *all* appear before the judgment seat of Christ,' says Paul to the Corinthians in his second letter (2 Cor. 5:10). This truth is confirmed in the closing chapters in the Book of Revelation, although using more colourful language:

> Then I saw a great white throne and him who was seated on it. The earth and the heavens fled from his presence, and there was no place for them. And I saw the dead, great and small, standing before the throne, and books were opened. Another book was opened, which is the book of life. The dead were judged according to what they had done as recorded in the books. The sea gave up the dead that were in it, and death and Hades gave up the dead that were in them, and each person was judged according to what they had done. Then death and Hades were thrown into the lake of fire. The lake of fire is the second death. Anyone whose name was not found written in the book of life was thrown into the lake of fire. (Rev. 20:11-15)

In these closing chapters of Revelation, Christians do not always agree on the exact nature of the final details. What, for example, is the second death mentioned towards the end of this passage? There can be, I believe, legitimate disagreement on these matters, but the overall point being made here is clear: there is a general resurrection of all people (including Hades giving up her dead) following which there is judgment for all.

Unsurprisingly, sleep is not generally language that unbelievers use. Many (though not all) do not like to acknowledge the possibility of resurrection because it implies the possibility of an accounting. Those who do, often have some vague notion of 'being OK'. Those of us who have read God's word carefully, however, know that it is only in Christ that we will be able to stand with any confidence before the judgment throne of God.

And sleep – such a beautiful thing! – might seem a funny way to anticipate what the prophets called the 'great and dreadful day of the Lord' (for example, Mal. 4:5). But I hope you can see how appropriate it is. For we sleep soundly if we do not fear the next day.

I once appeared in an important court case as an expert witness. I had a bad first day in the stand. The prosecuting counsel did not warm to my testimony and the judge joined in with disbelief. I had the misfortune to follow a famous, knighted businessman whose testimony contradicted mine, and the court seemed more inclined to believe him than me.

That night I did not sleep. I was a wreck. The next day's evidence weighed heavily on my mind, not helped by the closing words of the judge who had told me to 'go home and consider very carefully what you have said on oath.' I felt like a naughty schoolboy being told off by the headmaster.

The anticipation of the next day meant that sleep eluded me.

Soon, however, the court case ended (we lost) and that was the end of that. I cannot tell you how well I slept! If we have nothing to worry about the next day, we know we are more inclined to sleep. And this is why sleep is such a good metaphor for *Christian* death (even though it is true for *all* death).

Sound sleep comes through having nothing to fear – we've seen that already. And it is true for death – death which has lost its sting because 'death has been swallowed up in victory' (1 Cor. 15:54). For the believer, death holds no terror. We know that the righteousness of Christ covers us. We know that though we are unable to stand before the judgment seat of God in our own standing, we do not have to do so. We stand in Christ, and therefore stand cleansed, forgiven, restored.

EVERYTHING WILL BE BETTER TOMORROW

And, in fact, that final sleep will see us gloriously awakened to a better life where our bodies are transformed. The Apostle Paul calls this 'home with the Lord'. It is the moment when we shall be clothed in our heavenly and eternal bodies.

> For we know that if the earthly tent we live in is destroyed, we have a building from God, an eternal house in heaven, not built by human hands. Meanwhile, we groan, longing to be clothed instead with our heavenly dwelling, because when we are clothed we will not be found naked.... Therefore we are always confident and

> know that as long as we are at home in the body
> we are away from the Lord....We are confident,
> I say, and would prefer to be away from the body
> and at home with the Lord. (2 Cor. 5:1-8)

I wonder if Christians should make more of this connection between sleep and death. It is not just that the nouns are almost interchangeable but, as we have begun to see, one is a picture of the other.

Perhaps you are reading this book and you don't share this confidence about what comes next. It is quite possible that you think of yourself in some Christian way, but you can't bring yourself to think about death as a kind of sleep. It all seems too frightening and too final. If so, I encourage you to think some more. Equating death with sleep is only possible if you know the reality of a forgiven life and what it means to be united with Christ Jesus, sharing with Him in His death *and* resurrection. This is the confidence of Paul, a confidence God promises to all who repent and believe in Him.

And it means that when Christians go to sleep we should be praying for a good night's rest, but also recognising that one glorious day we shall fall asleep to this world forever. It means that when we wake up and thank God for a good night's rest we should be thanking Him that one glorious day we will wake in His presence for all eternity.

It is quite possible that our world today understands this link better than it knows. Our culture's low view of sleep – as something which just interrupts the real business of the day – may be reflective of a low view of death: you've got to pack as much in before you're finished. We draw up 'bucket lists' – fifty things to do before you're fifty, for example. Our culture does not want to recognise that God gives us limitations and boundaries to life – both temporal (waking and sleeping) and eternal (life and death).

It goes without saying that Christians should think altogether differently.

And I wonder if it works both ways. Understanding that one day we will wake up in the presence of our Saviour makes treasuring sleep now an easier task. We know that – on that final day – we will wake up free from sorrows, pains, sickness and sin. There is a reason that those who fall asleep in Jesus can 'rest in peace' as some gravestones say. And so it should be with our earthly sleep. In God's goodness, He gives us sleep and it functions as a respite from the cares and worries of the world. As a friend of mine often says to me, 'everything will look better in the morning.' It is understanding the spiritual reality that will make our present sleep even more of a joy and tonic for our bodies and minds.

SING IT AGAIN

Remember that cemetery near where I live? As graves get more recent, the phrase 'asleep in Jesus' seems to have disappeared. It's not so popular now; it sounds rather saccharine and sentimental. But it should not be. It should be the longing of every believer – to fall asleep in Him, for we *know* we shall awake. There's a lovely old hymn which expresses this beautifully:

Asleep in Jesus! blessed sleep!
From which none ever wakes to weep;
a calm and undisturbed repose,
unbroken by the last of foes.

Asleep in Jesus! Oh, how sweet
to be for such a slumber meet;
with holy confidence to sing
that death has lost its painful sting!

Asleep in Jesus! peaceful rest!
Whose waking is supremely blest;
no fear, no woe, shall dim that hour
that manifests the Saviour's power.

Asleep in Jesus! Oh, for me
may such a blissful refuge be;
securely shall my ashes lie,
waiting the summons from on high.

Asleep in Jesus! Though far it seems
your kindred and their graves may be;
but there is still a blessed sleep,
from which none ever wakes to weep.

Margaret MacKay (1802-1887)[2]

Sleep is part of our created humanity, a good gift from God to be treasured and enjoyed; an earthly picture of a spiritual reality.

So, what should we think and do when this glorious gift eludes us?

---

2. A hymn by English hymn writer Margaret MacKay. It appeared first in *The Christian's Annual* published in 1832 and can be found in many Victorian hymn books.

5

Hope the bed bugs don't bite!

Answers to a good night's sleep

'Doctor! Doctor! I can't get to sleep!'
        'Well, lie on the edge of the bed and you'll soon drop off!'

This joke proves that the 'old ones' are certainly *not* the best. What is more, anyone who has ever struggled to sleep (and that includes me) will know that there is nothing remotely funny about it. In fact, quite the opposite. As we've already seen, prolonged sleeplessness can be very debilitating indeed.

There are lots of reasons why people cannot sleep. Some of these will be practical ones. Some will be medical. Others still will be spiritual. It is this last category I want to concentrate on and, indeed, is the purpose of this little book. But we cannot jump straight to that category without at least a little exploration of these other factors.

PRACTICAL ANSWERS TO A GOOD NIGHT'S SLEEP

Most married people will tell you that they have a preferred side of the bed: left or right. I must confess to being a little stranger: for if you asked me which side of the bed I prefer, I would always answer 'the window side'. And sure enough, in our twenty-two plus years of marriage, my preferred side of the bed has switched from left to right and back again, depending on the location of the window in our bedroom at the time.

Fresh air helps me sleep. You may think I am a little strange. Or even inconsistent – why not go the whole way and sleep out under the stars?! But the truth is that there are plenty of practical answers to the question of sleep. Some of these are general – they affect everybody. Some, like my open window, are curiously specific.

Sleep experts call these environmental factors or 'sleep hygiene'. They have nothing to do with carbon emissions, greenhouse gases or having a shower before bed, but rather are about the *setting* of your sleep. There are, in other words, practical things you can do to help you sleep better.

This is not a book about environmental sleep solutions (there are plenty of those already), but it is important for me to name a few and suggest some things you could try. Why? Because there is wisdom in the world. Our sovereign God allows even those who don't acknowledge Him to understand something of humanity and have the wisdom to fix things that go wrong.

You and I should be thankful for that every time a nurse sticks a hypodermic in our arm or we go under the surgeon's knife. It's what theologians call *common grace*: the world is not as bad as it could be and there is wisdom to be had from listening to the world.

First of all, there are some *general* things you can try to help you sleep.[1] Central to these is having some sort of regular routine. Go to bed – as far as you are able – at the same time each day. Wake up at roughly the same time, if you can. Interestingly, experts also recommend that you only use your internal alarm clock to wake you.

Yeah, right. Some of us have jobs! Not every suggestion has equal merit!

Regularity is important. Parents know this from bedtime stories with little ones. The same book (which can almost be recited off by heart) is often the one which will send dozy toddlers over the edge and into sleep. For many, Dr Seuss's *Sleep Book* is a favourite.[2]

Creatures are starting to think about rest.

Two Biffer-Baum birds are now building their nest.

They do it each night. And quite often I wonder

How they do this big job without making a blunder.

But that is their problem.

Not yours. And not mine.

---

1. These are all tips gleaned from www.signaturemd.com, the website for a leading U.S. 'concierge medicine service provider' i.e., a paid service. Nevertheless, their advice on sleep is robust and echoed elsewhere.

2. Dr Seuss, *Sleep Book* (London, U.K: HarperCollins, 2003).

The point is: They're going to bed.

And that's fine.

Many people have found that clock-watching hinders sleep. So if, like me, you need an alarm clock to help you get up in the morning, try turning it away from you at night so you can't see the dial. There are some other obvious tips. You should reduce your caffeine intake, indulge in regular exercise (but not before bedtime), not sleep on a full (or empty) stomach and keep your bedroom dark and quiet. A good mattress and bedding are essential.

I might add that familiarity also helps. If you spend a lot of your nights away travelling, it can often be difficult to sleep. A friend of mine takes his own duvet with him when he travels in the U.K. This is less mad than it sounds. One U.S. hotel chain built its reputation on offering exactly the same kind of room wherever you stayed: same bed, same curtains, same linen. They promised that when you woke up, you would not know which city you were in. Whilst to some that might sound a little dull, to other frequent travellers it was a godsend.

And switch off that phone early!

Experts say today's obsession with gadgetry is a significant factor in troubled sleep. Forty-two per cent of Generation Y (aged 19–29) and 52 per cent of Generation Z (13–18) use their phones before going to bed for the night. Baby Boomers (48–64) should not be self-righteous. They fare little better, it's just that their gadgets are bigger: 67 per cent watch television immediately before retiring.[3] Such intensive interaction makes your mind buzz and, though you may *feel* sleepy, it tends to inhibit sleep.

What is generally understood is that alcohol *doesn't* help you sleep. That may surprise you. People often think that a few beers before bed or a nightcap whisky will help you nod off. That much – at least – is true. But alcohol, sleep scientists believe, does *not* help you sleep soundly through the night. Alcohol may help you *get* to sleep, but is also more likely to wake you in the middle of the night.

> Alcohol reduces the amount of time it takes to fall asleep and promotes deeper sleep for two to three hours; however it also increases awakenings and stage 1 non-REM sleep in the second half of the night. When used on a sustained basis, it creates more problems than it alleviates.[4]

No, alcohol is not the panacea that many think it is.

However, and I offer this advice cautiously, sex *is*. According to the U.S. director of the Berman Center for Women's Sexual Health[5], sexual activity not only reduces stress (which aids sleep) but also releases the chemical oxytocin which aids sleepiness. As Christians, of course, we understand that this

---

3. Based on a study by the National Sleep Foundation, *The 2011 Sleep in America Poll*.

4. E.L. Hillstrom, writing in D. G. Benner, and P. C. Hill (editors) *Baker Encyclopedia of Psychology and Counseling* (Grand Rapids, U.S.A.: Baker Books, 1999).

5. Interviewed on NBC News 13 February 2006. Available to watch online.

advice must be understood of sex in its proper God-given context, that is, in marriage. Moreover, there may be times when bad sex or disappointing sex leaves us awake and miserable. Nevertheless – in general terms – this is a striking truth that most married couples can rejoice in.

Strange working hours need not preclude good sleep. In fact, such people are often sleep 'experts'. In our church, we have a number of people who work shift patterns. Some regularly work what we call unsocial hours – they are night-shift workers. Others work irregular patterns – doctors, nurses, paramedics, police officers, and people like that. They sometimes work nights, sometimes days, sometimes mixed rotas. It strikes me that these folk in our congregation often have some of the best solutions to get to sleep at irregular times. Perhaps you've got someone you know whose advice you could seek? When we ran a sleep seminar in our church, some of the best practical advice came from just such a worker.

Secondly, there may be more *specific* solutions that work for you but will not necessarily work for others. These are going to include my open-window theory. Beware of investing too much expectation in these kinds of solutions, however. If your friend offers you a sure-fire solution to your disturbed nights, it will not necessarily follow that what works for them works for you. Fresh air works for me, but it may just make you chilly and miserable.

You'll find many more suggestions on websites set up by organisations such as the U.K.'s National

Health Service[6] and the U.S. National Sleep Foundation[7]. Be aware, however, that some sites are sponsored by, or simply marketing tools for, mattress manufacturers. This doesn't make them worthless (many contain good advice), but it is worth knowing who is supplying your information.

MEDICAL ANSWERS TO A GOOD NIGHT'S SLEEP[8]
I'm no doctor, and this is not meant to be a medical book. Nevertheless, it's important to recognise that, if you have trouble sleeping, the problems may well be medical. In this book, I've tried to show that, just as sleep is a good gift from our Father in heaven, so sleeplessness may require spiritual remedies. However, it may also be important for you to get medical help if your problem is primarily a physical or psychological one.

There are some very obvious physical reasons why sleep may not be easy. If you suffer from a bad back or other kind of chronic pain, for example, you may regularly experience disturbed nights. If you have a cold and, therefore, trouble breathing easily, sleep may also be elusive. Some physical complaints are longer-term. Sleep apnoea is a condition where your breathing stops for brief spells whilst you are asleep, thus waking you up momentarily. It's not dangerous as such, but it will make you tired the next day and can increase the risk of cardiovascular disease. The National Health Service in the U.K.

---

6. http://www.nhs.uk/livewell/insomnia/pages/insomniatips.aspx, accessed 31 December 2013.

7. www.sleepfoundation.org.

8. I'm grateful to Dr Rebecca Scott, a local GP (family doctor), for her help in putting together this brief section.

estimates that it affects 4 per cent of middle-aged men and 2 per cent of middle-aged women.[9]

Certain kinds of medication, for example, anti-depressants, beta blockers, steroids, thyroxine (thyroid treatment) and some asthma treatments (sympathomimetics, like the asthma drug salbutamol) can also distort sleep patterns. It should also perhaps be obvious that drug and substance abuse and over-use can contribute to sleeplessness. We all know that drinking coffee before bedtime is unlikely to send us off to sleep quickly.

Serious physical conditions also disturb our sleep – these include heart problems, asthma, Alzheimer's, Parkinson's disease, arthritis and gastro-intestinal/urinary issues. Many of these are more likely to affect older people, though not exclusively so.

However, sleep difficulties can also be caused by psychological factors. These take many forms, can be incredibly complex and have various degrees of seriousness. It is worth outlining just a few to show the variety of issues that may cause trouble.[10]

Psychosocial stressors are usually short-term and include situational stress (for example, worry about employment or finances), environmental stress (perhaps noise) and one-off issues such as the death of someone close. As we shall see in just a moment, there may be spiritual issues at stake here.

Psychiatric disorders often affect sleep. These include mood disorders such as depression, bipolar

---

9.   NHS Choices website. www.nhs.uk.

10.   This information is taken from the NICE (National Institute for Health and Care Excellence) Clinical Knowledge Summary: Insomnia. http://cks.nice.org.uk/insomnia#!topicsummary, accessed 31 December 2013.

disorder and dysthymia (a milder but longer-lasting depression). Anxiety disorders are another obvious cause for sleeplessness and may include panic attacks or post-traumatic stress disorder. More serious still are psychotic illnesses such as paranoia, schizophrenia and delusions.

Just because you cannot sleep doesn't mean you have one of these – but it is always worth checking out with your doctor, and the good news is that clinicians are well trained in spotting and treating all of these illnesses.

Of course, this common-grace advice can only go so far. The world will not tell you that there may be biblical and spiritual answers to sleeplessness. But there are. And, even if you suffer medically, understanding and addressing spiritual answers to sleeplessness may still help. So, that's where we turn to now.

BIBLICAL ANSWERS TO A GOOD NIGHT'S SLEEP
Given that the Bible has so much to say about sleep and its significance, it's not surprising that it also suggests some reasons why we find it hard to sleep. What follows is not an exhaustive list and – as I've pointed out several times (I want to make sure you hear this) – there may be medical (physical and mental) or environmental reasons why sleep is hard to come by.

But, I don't think sleep is at any time *less* than a spiritual issue. Let me explain. Our beings cannot easily be separated into physical and spiritual elements. We are whole beings. Even very straightforward physical ailments have spiritual elements and significance to them.

For example, let's say I broke my arm badly. I did this once, on the way to Anglican confirmation classes, as it happens. My arm was in plaster for several months. It was my right arm and I could not write, play the piano or take part in tennis. I had to learn to use my left hand.

Now, that was a purely physical issue, wasn't it? My arm was broken in several places, my wrist was damaged and it just needed time and good medical care to sort it out.

Right.

Well, sort of right.

There's no indication that there was anything deeply spiritual going on behind the injury. It might have been a sign I should be a Baptist and not an Anglican, perhaps. But certainly nothing more. I don't think I tripped and fell because of some unresolved sin at that particular moment.

However, here's the thing: how I reacted to that injury *was* a spiritual issue: how I dealt with the disappointment of a promising tennis career wrecked (at least that's how I think of it now!); how I coped with the worry of falling behind in school because I couldn't write; how I kept my spirits up and my Christian joy intact; how I would serve in church playing the piano with only one hand... The list goes on and on.

It was a physical issue which needed medical treatment and resolution. But it would be naïve to say that it had no spiritual resolution. Similarly, someone suffering from an anxiety disorder may be given various forms of treatment by the doctor, but these will include thinking through how information is processed by the patient: there will always be Christian wisdom which needs to be brought to bear on such solutions.

So, there may well be medical reasons for your struggle with sleep. These may be very complex and difficult mental health issues, for example, that take a lot of sorting. However, there will still be spiritual elements to address. I'm not suggesting that everything on my list below will apply to you. Most probably, if your sleep problems are medical or environmental, these answers may seem a bit simplistic.

However, I want to encourage you to read on anyway. If nothing else, understanding that it is ultimately our sovereign God who gives sleep to His children, should inform your prayers and those of people who are supporting you.

One of my daughters, who has herself struggled with sleep, has given me some wise advice on this very subject. She tells me that, even if your problem is not fundamentally spiritual, thinking Christianly is a help. Christians ought to be encouraged by what the Bible says about sleep. It assists you to view sleep positively and, even when you don't find sleep easy, to – at the very least – make the most of times of rest.

Solution 1: Ask God for sleep
If sleep is a gift, then it may simply be that we need to ask the Giver for it.

You may think that is very, very simplistic. However, the testimony of Scripture is that we sometimes do not receive things because we do not ask for them. When James is writing to the scattered Christians under his care, he reminds them (squabbling as they are) that they may be pursuing the wrong procedures.

> What causes fights and quarrels among you? Don't they come from your desires that battle within you? You desire but you do not have, so you kill. You covet but you cannot get what you want, so you quarrel and fight. You do not have because you do not ask God. When you ask, you do not receive, because you ask with wrong motives, that you may spend what you get on your pleasures. (James 4:1-3)

There's some serious stuff going on in the churches to whom James is writing! But the principles cross over the centuries. There is disagreement in church life because desires are misplaced. People don't have what they want, and they see others doing better. Some don't ask God. Others do, but their motives are to be like those who have more. It's all a recipe for disaster.

We can learn a couple of things. First, it is right to ask the Giver for His good gifts. Earlier in his letter, James has described God in just this way: 'Every good and perfect gift is from above, coming down from the Father of the heavenly lights, who does not change like shifting shadows.' (James 1:17). James is trying to encourage his readers who are facing dreadful difficulties. Those temptations don't come from God. However, God is not passive either. He gives good and perfect gifts.

If sleep – as we have seen – is a gift, we should not be ashamed to ask for it. Our heavenly Father knows what we need before we ask Him (Matt. 6:8) and so it should be natural for us to pray for sleep as part of our daily bread (Matt. 6:11). It seems to me that this is a strange omission from the prayers of many Christians.

Second, it may well be that our prayers for sleep are unanswered because we've asked with wrong motives. We must entertain that possibility, mustn't we? James points out that it is possible to ask 'with wrong motives'.

What might those wrong motives be? In James 4, the wrong motive stems from covetousness – wanting what others have. To be honest, that may seem to be a common feeling for those who struggle with sleep. However, it is helpful to be clear about coveting. Coveting is wanting something for yourself that rightly belongs to someone else. Coveting your neighbour's house is wanting his house for yourself. Coveting your neighbour's wife or his servant or his donkey (all part of the tenth commandment) is wishing that a particular possession of your friend were actually yours.

In that sense, I don't think many of us covet the sleep of others. I don't think to myself, I wish that I could take Bill's sleep and have it for myself (and that he would no longer have it). Looking at Bill and seeing his sleep and saying 'I wish I could sleep too' is not a sin; it is not a breaking of the tenth commandment. Sleep, remember, is a good gift.

But it is, I would suggest, possible to ask for sleep for the wrong motives. This is more subtle, perhaps, than the presenting issue in James, but still a temptation nevertheless. Remember, sleep is a good gift, and if we are asking for it from the Creator-Giver so that we might enjoy the benefits it conveys, there is surely nothing wrong in that! The tired mum who craves sleep so she can serve her children well the following day without being cross with them is right to cry out for sleep! It's more than OK to pray that sort of prayer.

What, then, might wrong motives be? In the Lord's Prayer, Jesus teaches His disciples to pray 'Give us today our daily bread' (Matt. 6:11). Bread is a very ordinary daily requirement and implicit within this prayer is the idea that we pray to God for what we need and *nothing more*. We don't ask God for a daily banquet, for example. So, it must be true that a demand to God which moves outside those boundaries looks remarkably like asking with wrong motives. In other words, all our requests to our sovereign Father must be couched in terms of His gracious provision as the One who knows what we need.

And the gift ought to be accompanied by thankfulness! In Luke's Gospel, we read the story of Jesus healing the ten men with leprosy (Luke 17:11-19). It's a striking story as only one of the ten has the faith (that's the word Jesus uses) to come back and thank the Saviour for what He has done. 'Has no one returned to give praise to God except this foreigner?', He asks. The life of a Christian should be marked by thankfulness.

I'm not suggesting that God operates on a tit-for-tat basis. Jesus did not 'un-heal' the nine who did not return. Nevertheless, if we have understood sleep as a gift from our Father in heaven, our lives will be marked by a joyful thankfulness to the Giver of all good gifts.

Solution 2: It may be an issue of faith

Let me paint an extreme picture for you. It's based on a true story. Let's imagine you go to sleep in India at a friend's house. Earlier there had been an infestation of giant cockroaches – perhaps three or four inches across. You know they came in through the open window. But let's imagine that you're the kind of sleeper who likes the window to be open. You've got trouble. Unless you can securely fix some kind of screen across the window, the thought of those flying roaches is going to trouble you all night. But if there is a screen and you trust it, sleep will come much more easily.

You may have worked out from the energy of the illustration that this is more than something I dreamt up. It really happened. And yes, you'll be glad to know that the screen did its job. It was a bug-free night.

We've already seen how David's sleep was grounded in the knowledge that the LORD was watching over him. His security from his enemies (real people, not cockroaches) was not down to an army or a set of bodyguards but because he knew that 'you alone, LORD, make me dwell in safety' (Ps. 4:8). The LORD neither slumbers nor sleeps.

If we have a strong and secure knowledge of the sovereign hand of God upon us, it should help us sleep. Let me put it like this: as you lie down to sleep, nothing can happen to you that has not been sovereignly ordained by the Ruler of the universe. He knows all things. He sees all things. He plans all things. He 'works out everything in conformity with the purpose of his will' (Eph. 1:11).

That even includes death. If death comes to you this night, it is because He has numbered your days and you have reached your number. It even, can I say this reverently, applies to cockroaches!

In fact, we are quick to teach our nervous children this truth when they can't sleep. We glibly tell them that God is in control. They may be scared by a noise or a worry or a shadow. But, we say, God is looking over you. We might even say a version of that well-known prayer:

> Now I lay me down to sleep,
> I pray the Lord my soul to keep.
> Guide me safely through the night,
> Wake me with the morning light.

But do we believe it ourselves? Or, more likely, are we like the disciples in the boat, panicking through the storm? It's not right, I believe, to spiritualise that story for its primary meaning. It is not, first and foremost, a story about being calm in the calamities of life. But if Jesus is indeed the One who commands the wind and the waves, it must surely follow that being with Him is the supreme calming presence.

If my lack of sleep is linked to my being anxious or worried, then I am uncertain about the sovereign rule of God. Ultimately, like the disciples, this is an issue of faith. That's why Jesus commands His followers:

> Therefore, I tell you, do not worry about your life, what you will eat or drink; or about your body, what you will wear. Is not life more than food, and the body more than clothes? Look at the birds of the air; they do not sow or reap or store away in barns, and yet your heavenly Father feeds them. Are you not much more valuable then they? Can any one of you by worrying add a single hour to your life? (Matt. 6:25-27)

Jesus is clear (and the passage continues in the same vein). Worrying is wrong. It serves no practical purpose – it does not add an hour to your life; it also denies the sovereign provision of our Father who feeds the birds and will feed you too. On this basis, lying awake at night worrying about tomorrow is not simply a misuse of the sleeping hours, it is a downright denial of the provision of God.

It is worth being stark about this because we can often justify our anxiety. To be honest, there are many things for me to be anxious about: work, home, family, finances, the car (which constantly seems to break down)... like most people, the list is endless.

What is more, it's easy to get into a stew about some of these things. It's hard to see things clearly and rationally at night-time. Issues which are relatively minor loom large. We can often be guilty of adding speculation on speculation. What if the car breaks down? What if it breaks down whilst I'm on the way to an important meeting? What if I missed that meeting and was sacked? That sort of irrational way of thinking is a common enough occurrence when we are lying awake with nothing else to occupy our minds.

That was the reason for my sleepless night before my second court appearance. I see that now. My anxiety and concern were entirely misplaced. I was worried about what the judge might say to me; even if, as he threatened, he were to accuse me of perjury. And as I rolled from one side to another, these problems seemed to grow in importance and in the seriousness of the possible outcomes.

It's all nonsense. That's what I needed to tell myself. My soul needed a good talking-to. God is sovereign. Jesus is on the throne. His Spirit is in my heart.

If that kind of situation resonates with you, it might seem a little glib to say that the answer is faith. But that is the Bible answer. The Apostle Peter is clear that a right relationship with God, where a Christian casts himself upon the Lord, is the answer.

> Humble yourselves, therefore, under God's mighty hand, that he may lift you up in due time. Cast all your anxiety on him because he cares for you. (1 Pet. 5:6-7)

Do you see that the command to cast your worries upon the Lord is linked closely to walking humbly before Him? We often quote the second part of this couplet without the important first part. A humble heart before God which lays before Him all its troubles and concerns is the sign of deep faith, a faith that will help us sleep.

How do we go about getting such faith? Is faith something we can just 'do' or 'do more'? Hardly; it is a gift from God (Eph. 2:8). I'm convinced that – as our verse from 1 Peter hints – the answer to a lack of faith is to humble ourselves before the One who is supremely faithful. In fact, 'Faithful' is His name! (Rev. 19:11). Meditating on the faithfulness of our sovereign God is the way to shift our thinking from me and my flaky faith to the One who is always and ever faithful in all He does.

And for those who are worried about death, sleep is the great gift. It reminds you that death is not the end, and so death is not something to be anxious about. Trusting in Christ Jesus, you can sleep soundly knowing that if this is your time, a greater awakening awaits.

Solution 3: You may need to learn contentment
Closely linked to this issue of trust is the question of contentment. Sleep, or rather the lack of it, is often deeply connected to anxiety. This is true medically (as we briefly saw). But it is also true spiritually (as we've also just seen).

The flip side of lacking in trust is that we need to learn Christian contentment. One of my favourite books on my shelf is a Puritan book based on lectures given at a church just around the corner from where I live. The lectures were given early in the morning before folk in the church went to work. The congregation was hungry to hear their lecturer (his official title). His name was Jeremiah Burroughs, and I know the book so well I only have to look at its spine to be both challenged and warmed. The title of the book is *The Rare Jewel of Christian Contentment* and I heartily commend either it or one of its modern versions.[11]

Contentment is a godly virtue and is best expressed by the Apostle Paul: 'I have learned to be content whatever the circumstances' (Phil. 4:11). Paul goes on to say how those circumstances include all kinds of extremes: 'in need....in plenty...well fed...hungry...in plenty...in want'.

Contentment is, of course, a consequence of a belief and trust in the sovereign provision of our Father, who gives us what we need. However, it is more precise than my previous injunction. We worry about many things and about how circumstances may turn out. But contentment is that settled comfort Christians have in knowing that God knows what we need, in the greatest detail.

For myself, I am only too aware that this is a godly characteristic I need to keep asking God to grant to me and nurture in me. The reality is that we are truly fighting against the world in this area, because the world is constantly trying to convince

---

11. Jeremiah Burroughs, *The Rare Jewel of Christian Contentment* (Edinburgh, U.K.: The Banner of Truth Trust, 1964). A good modern version picking up on this and the writing of Thomas Boston is: William Barcley, *The Secret of Contentment* (Phillipsburg, U.S.A.: P&R Books, 2010).

us that we don't have enough of anything. That's the whole point of advertising, after all.

Contentment, therefore, is our weapon against the world's assault of 'more, more, more'. And if that desire for more is what keeps you awake, then contentment is what you need.

There is a hint of this in the book of Ecclesiastes.

> The sleep of a labourer is sweet,
> whether they eat little or much,
> but as for the rich, their abundance
> permits them no sleep. (Eccles. 5:12)

Solomon's words may be interpreted two ways. He may mean that if you work hard, you will sleep well. A day's manual labour is great for getting you off to sleep (and this is advice some people ought to take on board!).

However, in the context, it is probably better to understand Solomon's words slightly differently. He paints the labourer in contrast not to the lazy man, but to the rich man. 'Their abundance permits them no sleep.' In other words, he is always thinking about *more* – how to make *more*, earn *more*, keep *more*. As Solomon has only just said, 'Whoever loves money never has enough; whoever loves wealth is never satisfied with their income.' (Eccles. 5:10).

The hand-to-mouth labourer who is paid his wage at the end of the day has no such worries. As such, I believe this is a proverb about contentment.

And contentment is key to a good night's sleep. Ultimately, argues Burroughs, this means seeing that the mercies that we have in Christ (he means our salvation) outweigh any other consideration. To put it in the language of the bedroom, if we go to sleep as Christians, we go to sleep as having everything. There is nothing that the world can give us to fill us up or complete us – we are complete already. Perhaps you need to learn that kind of contentment?

Solution 4: You may need to give up idols

We saw back in a previous chapter how it is possible to love sleep so much that it displaces God's rightful place. I don't think many people will find that surprising. It is a temptation we face with any of God's good gifts. In their rightful place, they are gifts to be enjoyed and treasured, but it is quite possible to take the best things God gives and elevate them above Christ. Perhaps this is what Paul means by those whose 'god is their stomach' (Phil. 3:19).

U.S. pastor-teacher Tim Keller has helpfully written on the subject of idolatry to show how much of sin can be understood in this category. I don't believe it is the only Bible category for sin (it also has much to say about law breaking). Nevertheless, it is a helpful model. What do we put before Christ in our love and affections?

Some put families first. Families are obviously good and worthy, delightful even. Others put work. Again a good thing. For others still, it is sex or money. And so the list goes on. And for some, I would suggest, it may be sleep. This may be especially true if you lack it. We do not make idols only of the things we have, but also of the things we don't have.

Making sleep an idol may be a temptation both for those who sleep well *and* for those who do not. 'Do not love sleep or you will grow poor; stay awake and you will have food to spare' (Prov. 20:13). The proverb here is really about working hard. If you love sleep so much that you never get out of bed to work, you're going to be as poor as a church mouse, and as hungry too.

Nevertheless, the warning not to 'love sleep' stands. As Christians, we always ought to be checking our hearts to make sure we are not putting the good gift before the Giver.

Perhaps this is an idol you need to release?

Solution 5: There may be an issue to resolve

I promised we would return to Psalm 77 and here we do. Psalm 77 is a psalm of Asaph, leader of the temple musicians in the time of King David (1 Chron. 16:5). The song describes the process by which he moves from crisis through to deep trust. It is a painful journey, beginning, as it does, with some words which will ring true for many believers.

> [1]I cried out to God for help;
> I cried out to God to hear me.
> [2]When I was in distress, I sought the LORD;
> at night I stretched out untiring hands,
> and I would not be comforted.
> [3]I remembered you, God, and I groaned;
> I meditated, and my spirit grew faint.
> [4]You kept my eyes from closing;
> I was too troubled to speak.
> [5]I thought about the former days,

the years of long ago;
[6]I remembered my songs in the night.
My heart meditated and my spirit asked:
[7]'Will the LORD reject for ever?
Will he never show his favour again?
[8]Has his unfailing love vanished for ever?
Has his promise failed for all time?
[9]Has God forgotten to be merciful?
Has he in anger withheld his compassion?'

The exact nature of the crisis is not simple: some commentators see it as a straightforward issue of faith – Asaph begins by doubting but is brought round. Others see the opening verses as a divinely ordained appointment for Asaph to feel the burden of the state of the nation. Either way, Asaph's words ring true for those who struggle to sleep.

And either way, the shock of the psalm is that it is the Giver of sleep, the LORD God Himself, who keeps Asaph awake. His eyes are kept from closing. To cut a long story short, the issue is resolved. Ultimately, it is Asaph's meditation on the Exodus – *the* salvation event of the Old Testament – which restores his outlook.

And whether you think this is Asaph wrestling with his doubt or you see Asaph being given a divine concern for the state of God's people, the remedy is the same. God, the good Giver of sleep, keeps Asaph awake so that Asaph will be in tune with the divine melody.

This is a remarkable truth. It means, quite simply, that we sometimes need to ask the question 'why?' when sleep evades us. Our lack of sleep –

painful as it is (and Asaph's description is nothing if not painful) – may be a divine appointment to sort something out.

Our sovereign God may be using our waking to teach us a truth, give us a burden or – and this is perhaps the least comfortable option – cause us to address a sin. None of these should be written off. I'm not saying this is definitely *why* you are not sleeping! But biblically, we would have to say, it may have something to do with it. What is God teaching you in the sleepless hours?

There is perhaps a hint of this in David's own psalm of testimony in Psalm 6.

> ⁴Turn, LORD, and deliver me;
> save me because of your unfailing love.
> ⁵Among the dead no one proclaims your name.
> Who praises you from his grave?
> ⁶I am worn out from my groaning.
> All night long I flood my bed with weeping
> and drench my couch with tears.
> ⁷My eyes grow weak with sorrow;
> they fail because of all my foes.
> ⁸Away from me, all you who do evil,
> for the LORD has heard my weeping.
> ⁹The LORD has heard my cry for mercy;
> the LORD accepts my prayer.
> ¹⁰All my enemies will be overwhelmed with shame
> and anguish;
> they will turn back and suddenly be put to shame.

Put simply, David's struggle with his enemies keeps him awake. He needs to learn that the covenant

God protects His covenant king. The king's prayer will be heard because of the LORD's faithfulness to His covenant. That is where David ends up – but he needs a sleepless night to get there.

Perhaps we can dwell on this solution for too long. But it may also be one which Christians are loath to consider. It may be that your sleeplessness is a sign that the covenant-keeping and saving Lord of all wants to do business with you.

We see that wonderfully illustrated in the book of Esther. The story of Queen Esther is a terrific story, full of pace and excitement and it all turns on one particular event – the inability of the king to sleep. 'That night the king could not sleep; so he ordered the book of the chronicles, the record of his reign, to be brought and read to him.' (Esther 6:1). It is this one night that leads to the honour of Mordecai and the eventual downfall of his enemy, Haman. And it all begins with a rather restless night.

I believe it's good to think of sleeplessness in terms of what God is doing. He is sovereign over all our comings and goings, sleepings and wakings. So to ignore what He might be showing us in sleeplessness is worse than casual. It is a denial of His universal rule.

There is, in other words, another kind of contentment to learn. It is that when God, in His providence, does keep our eyes from closing, we need to be able to say that He knows what He is doing. We need to be able to honestly cry out, 'What are you teaching me, O Lord?' This is as much a contentment as the ability to go to sleep free from worry about the cares of the day.

So, sleep is part of our created humanity, a good gift from God to be treasured and enjoyed; an earthly picture of a spiritual reality. Sleeplessness is troublesome, but not unfixable and sometimes even necessary for our sanctification. Spiritual problems need spiritual answers and I commend to you some reflection on some of these possible solutions.

A WORD TO NEW PARENTS

My wife and I have three children ourselves and twenty nieces and nephews. My wife's first niece was born when she was thirteen. The latest was born last week. We seem to have spent most of our dating and married life around newborns. So we have experienced something ourselves of the sleeping pressures that a baby brings into the house.

The reality is that all babies sleep a lot. Even when it doesn't seem like it. However, some sleep better than others. And some have sleep patterns more suitable to our own than others. For some new parents – and especially, may I say, new mums – the pressure of sleeplessness that comes from having a new baby in the house can be intense. The baby can drop off to sleep on an afternoon stroll. It's not so easy for mum, especially if there are other kids to be collected or looked after.

What's the answer to this particular problem? And does the Bible have any light to bear? The answer is no. And yes.

The Bible has nothing directly to say about sleep relating to babies and their parents over and above what we've already seen. But it does have something to say about the environment in which children are reared. In the New Testament, this environment has a name and it is called the church. This is more significant than you may imagine.

If a new mum is struggling to sleep because baby always seems to be awake, then help should be on hand from both dad *and* the church family. There should be a responsibility to care for one another in church; that kind of care is biblical and must surely include looking after the sleep-deprived. Perhaps it means someone picking up the other kids from school to allow mum to have an afternoon snooze? Perhaps it means doing an evening stint for a couple armed with a bottle of milk, ready to feed little Timmy.

And please remember, these *are* seasons. Seasons of parenting come and go remarkably quickly. It hardly seems possible that our eldest daughter is almost twenty. I still remember the stork delivering her.

It's true, disturbed sleep can continue to be a pattern for parents. Children who wake in the night often need the comfort of a mum or dad. They are not always able simply to tell themselves 'it was nothing' and go straight back to sleep. Such is the responsibility of parenting. These are real issues, painful too for those experiencing them.

Like the practical advice above, there is lots of wise counsel and help available from health professionals for those who find themselves in these situations. But this reality must not detract from the biblical riches we have unearthed in this little volume.

AND A WORD TO SLEEPY CHURCHGOERS

Perhaps the best-known sleep story in the Bible is found in the book of Acts. Paul is in Troas, where he is briefly stopping over as part of a longer trip. Not surprisingly, the believers there are eager to meet him.

> On the first day of the week we came together to break bread. Paul spoke to the people and, because he intended to leave the next day, kept on talking until midnight. There were many lamps in the upstairs room where we were meeting. Seated in a window was a young man named Eutychus, who was sinking into a deep sleep as Paul talked on and on. When he was sound asleep, he fell to the ground from the third storey and was picked up dead. Paul went down, threw himself on the young man and put his arms around him. 'Don't be alarmed,' he said. 'He's alive!' Then he went upstairs again and broke bread and ate. After talking until daylight, he left. The people took the young man home alive and were greatly comforted. (Acts 20:7-12)

Isn't this a great story! It gives hope to everyone who falls asleep in church, though I must caution you (if that is your temptation) to avoid open windows. Commentators sometimes disagree over exactly why young Eutychus fell asleep. Perhaps he was bored? It was, after all, a very, very long sermon. Perhaps the many lamps gave off fumes which made him sleepy? Possibly – it's a strange inclusion in the text if it doesn't have some significance.

However, in purely matter-of-fact terms we can say what the text says, which is that he fell asleep and fell out of the window, dead. Thankfully, this was not the final sleep for him. Paul raised him from the dead and, in what must count as something of an understatement, 'the people....were greatly comforted.'

Here's the point to make. This passage, glorious though it is, does not excuse falling asleep in church. I am a preacher. I count it a great privilege to study and pray during the week and bring God's Word to His people Sunday by Sunday. And it saddens me, therefore, to sometimes see people asleep. Acts 20 is not included in the Bible to permit such reckless behaviour.

And I do believe it is reckless. As Christians (and I sit in the pew too), we should do whatever it takes to make ourselves ready to meet Christ Jesus in His Word. There may be many reasons why we might nod off – perhaps an illness? But if it is tiredness, it seems to me that is hardly commendable! An earlier night is what the spiritual doctor would order.

Take heart, however. Such wrongdoing is forgivable. Just as Eutychus was raised from the dead, so we too can find forgiveness if this is our persistent and besetting problem! But it *is* a problem that needs fixing.

6

FEELING SLEEPY NOW?

It has never been my intention to send you to sleep with this book. However, I have tried to show you what the Bible says about sleep and hope, therefore, in some way, to make sleep easier for you.

However, ultimately – as we have seen – it's God who gives good sleep. Sleep is His good gift, part of our created humanity. It's a gift to be treasured and enjoyed. I hope you feel more thankful for the sleep you do enjoy. I trust that you will be more appreciative when you wake up in the morning. I have certainly learnt to be.

But, most importantly, I trust that you will have learnt to eagerly look forward to that day when the old order of things will pass away and when our sleep will not just prepare us for the next day but for eternity. One day sleep will come and we will wake up in the presence of our glorious Saviour forever.

Perhaps this old Puritan prayer will help. It is taken from *The Valley of Vision*, a wonderful little book of old prayers and is reproduced here with the kind permission of the publisher.[1]

SLEEP

Blessed Creator, thou hast promised thy beloved sleep;

Give me restoring rest needful for tomorrow's toil;

If dreams be mine, let them not be tinged with evil.

Let thy Spirit make my time of repose a blessed temple of his holy presence.

May my frequent lying down make me familiar with death,

the bed I approach remind me of the grave,

the eyes I now close picture to me their final closing.

Keep me always ready, waiting for admittance to thy presence.

Weaken my attachment to earthly things.

May I hold life loosely in my hand,

knowing that I receive it on condition of its surrender;

As pain and suffering betoken transitory health,

may I not shrink from a death that introduces me to the freshness of eternal youth.

I retire this night in full assurance of one day awaking with thee.

---

1. Arthur Bennett (Ed.), *The Valley of Vision* (Edinburgh, UK: The Banner of Truth Trust, 1975), p. 298, and reproduced here with the kind permission of the publisher.

All glory for this precious hope,

for the gospel of grace,

for thine unspeakable gift of Jesus,

for the fellowship of the Trinity.

Withhold not thy mercies in the night season;

Thy hand never wearies,

thy power needs no repose,

thine eye never sleeps.

Help me when I helpless lie,

when my conscience accuses me of sin,

when my mind is harassed by foreboding thoughts,

when my eyes are held awake by personal anxieties.

Show thyself to me as the God of all grace, love
    and power;

Thou hast a balm for every wound,

a solace for all anguish,

a remedy for every pain,

a peace for all disquietude.

Permit me to commit myself to thee awake or asleep.

Growing up, I remember watching the children's TV programme *The Magic Roundabout*. Each episode ended the same way, with Zebedee calling all the characters to order. 'Time for bed', he would say.

And when it is time, may your sleep truly be sweet.

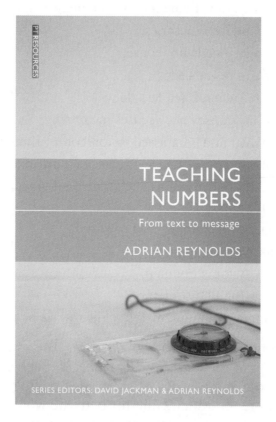

TEACHING
NUMBERS

From text to message

ADRIAN REYNOLDS

SERIES EDITORS: DAVID JACKMAN & ADRIAN REYNOLDS

ISBN 978-1-78191-156-3

Teaching Numbers
From Text to Message
ADRIAN REYNOLDS

God Speaks! The Book of Numbers follows the Journey of the Israelite people between the Exodus from Egypt and their entrance into the Promised Land. This book is deeply relevant for a wandering generation today who need to make their way back to God. The book points to Christ and provides important instruction for believers today. Discover how God speaks even in the wilderness!

Adrian has blessed us with a volume that is lively, solid and well-applied.

Sam Allberry
Assistant Pastor, St Marys, Author of *Lifted and Is God Anti-gay?*
Maidenhead, England

The Teaching series is a great resource for Bible study leaders and pastors, indeed for any Christian who wants to understand their Bible better.

Mark Dever
Senior Pastor of Capitol Hill Baptist Church and President of 9Marks.org, Washington, DC

This teaching series, written by skilled and trustworthy students of God's word, helps us to understand the Bible, believe it and obey it. I commend it to all Bible readers, but especially those whose task it is to teach the inspired word of God.

Peter Jensen
Archbishop of Sydney

Adrian Reynolds is Director of Ministry of the Proclamation Trust and also serves as associate minister at East London Tabernacle Baptist Church.